The Mirror Therapy

The Mirror Therapy

A Complete mind, body spiritual workout.
It will bring extraordinary gifts to your life!

by

Marcela Insignares

DORRANCE PUBLISHING CO., INC.
PITTSBURGH, PENNSYLVANIA 15222

The contents of this work including, but not limited to, the accuracy of events, people, and places depicted; opinions expressed; permission to use previously published materials included; and any advice given or actions advocated are solely the responsibility of the author, who assumes all liability for said work and indemnifies the publisher against any claims stemming from publication of the work.

All Rights Reserved
Copyright © 2006 by Marcela Insignares
No part of this book may be reproduced or transmitted in any form or by any means, electronic or mechanical, including photocopying, recording, or by any information storage and retrieval system without permission in writing from the publisher.

ISBN-10: 0-8059-6992-6
ISBN-13: 978-0-8059-6992-4

Printed in the United States of America

First Printing

For information or to order additional books, please write:
Dorrance Publishing Co., Inc.
701 Smithfield Street
Third Floor
Pittsburgh, Pennsylvania 15222-3906
U.S.A.
1-800-788-7654
Or visit our web site and on-line catalog at www.dorrancepublishing.com

*In memory of my dear father-in-law,
Saul Insignares Melo*

Author's Note

It is not my intention to prevent, treat, or cure any specific condition. You should seek professional help if you have any physical or mental problem. This book is not a substitute for medical advice. I am not responsible for the effects that come from following the exercises presented in this book.

Contents

Author's Note vii
Acknowledgments xi
My Little Gift to the World xiii
Who Am I? xv
Introduction xvii

Part I: The Mirror Therapy: Integrating Body, Mind, And Soul
Chapter 1: The Magic of Mirrors 3
Chapter 2: Loosing Our Will 5
Chapter 3: Transforming Lives 7
Chapter 4: Inspiring You 11
Chapter 5: My Story, The Foundation
   of the Mirror Therapy 13
Chapter 6: Developing the Mirror Therapy,
   Creating the Structure 21

Part II: Creating Your Routine
Chapter 1: What Is the Real Meaning
   of the Mirror Therapy? 27
Chapter 2: The Elements 29
Chapter 3: The Techniques 33
Chapter 4: Benefits 39
Chapter 5: My Favorite Quotes 41

References 47

Acknowledgments

To God, for inspiring me and giving me the knowledge and the experiences that I needed to make possible this project; to my parents, for giving me the opportunities and the education to succeed in life; to my dear husband, Saul, for his support and patience; to my children, Nicolas and Sebastian, for their great energy and optimism; and to my friend Mell, for her endless enthusiasm.

My Little Gift to the World

This book is for everybody—or at least for all those who need a little spark in their lives. It is a healing book which will help you to appreciate the simplicity of life in a complicated world. It is written in very simple, everyday language—easy to read, easy to understand, easy to enjoy! It is for refreshing, renewal, and soothing comfort; it will help you to nurture your being, catching the rhythm of Mother Nature and, of course, the divine rhythm of God, being in totally harmony and peace.

Who Am I?

I'm nobody, and I'm everybody.
I'm a messenger.
I'm a healer.
I'm a teacher.
I'm a student.
I'm a wife.
I'm a mother.
I'm a daughter.
I'm a sister.
I'm a friend.
I'm a neighbor.
I'm a human being.
I'm an ordinary woman who wants to help ordinary people to live extraordinary lives!

Introduction

If you are looking for a miracle—or at least for something that could change your life in a very positive way, bringing happiness and peace to your heart—*The Mirror Therapy* could be the answer to your prayers.

The Mirror Therapy is a routine I developed when I was going through a very difficult time in my life. I was completely lost and out of control, and I knew I needed something that could help me to recover my balance and give me the strength, peace of mind, and joy that I needed to live a great life.

Like many people, I was looking for quick fixes and easy answers to the difficult questions and adversities I faced in my life. I was overwhelmed with the endless options and information that the outside was giving me until I understood that the only way to regain control over my life was to search for my true "self." I really felt obligated to reach deeper, to come back to my self in a different manner in order to find the right answers to my complex questions and my inquiring mind.

For some divine reason I felt inspired to develop a routine I called the Mirror Therapy. It was the result of many years of soul searching, opening up a spiritual dimension that I had never before experienced. I do really believe that we are extremely intelligent and powerful beings, we just need to follow our inner-guide system to be able to develop our creativity, exploring, discovering, and finally knowing ourselves more fully.

Like many other disciplines, the Mirror Therapy is about self-transformation. It is the path to discovering the wisdom within you; connecting mind, body, and soul; keeping yourself in perfect balance. It is not a secret that we all possess an inner guidance system that shows us our path in everything, and I do really think that simple routines can help us to connect with it.

My purpose with this book is to help you to create your own routine—in other words, your own Mirror Therapy—based on your needs and circumstances. We are unique beings, and nobody can live our lives. It is our responsibility to take care of ourselves, and we have to accept this responsibility for our state of well being.

You will develop a routine just for you; it will be a personal experience You will be the designer, the architect, the creator of something that you will use as a part of your life. It will be a healthy habit, something that will help you to bring the real person out, something that will connect you with your higher self, and something that will allow you to recover the identity that has been stolen from you by a controlling world. You will find yourself permanently transformed, empowered physically, mentally, and spiritually.

I will be your guide, helping you through education, giving you information, and presenting my own personal experience as an example of someone who created an incredible discipline which turned to be the best gift ever.

I truly believe that if you look inside yourself you will find exactly what you need to live a great, joyful, and balanced life. I promise you will be amazed by the results. Be prepared for an incredible journey that will challenge your own capabilities—a journey that will bring magic to your life and will give you the opportunity to be in control again.

Part I
Integrating Body, Mind, and Soul

Chapter 1
The Magic of Mirrors

"The nature of the mind is like a mirror which has the natural and inherent capacity to reflect whatever is set before it, whether beautiful or ugly; but these reflections in no way affect or modify the nature of the mirror. It is the same with the state of contemplation: There is nothing to correct or alter or modify. What the practitioner does when entering into contemplation is simply to discover him in the condition of the mirror."
　Namkhai Norbu
　　Self-liberation through Seeing with Naked Awareness

In my quest for the miracle cure to my suffering, I discovered the magical power of mirrors. I can say that, although they were part of my everyday life, I never thought they were going to be a great tool that would help me to develop a routine that could change my life forever.

　I used to spend hours in front of mirrors when I was younger. I was obsessed with physical beauty, always trying to look better and trying to get the perfect look or the "ideal" image—according to the "out-world," in other words, magazines and television shows. Sometimes, frankly, I was really afraid of mirrors because the only things I could see were my imperfections. I remember complaining all the time about my body and doing extreme things to achieve the physical perfection I wanted.

Marcela Insignares

I used to work-out every day in front of mirrors at the gym or in my house, and it was as if I needed them for some reason. I needed to see the reflection of my body, although I was not really happy with the things I was seeing. One day, however, I discovered that those mirrors were reflecting my self, and that reflection was really "me." For some reason, that magical day I could go beyond my skin, my physical body, and feel for the first time a sense of profound unity within myself and with the outside world. What a mystical experience! I felt for the first time that my body was no longer a solid object in a material world but more like a manifestation of some kind of divine energy.

There was definitely something more deep and magical about those mirrors; there was something else in that reflection. It was like there were hidden messages that I could not see before, messages that I had to reveal sooner or later if I wanted to know who I really was. I discovered a magical bridge which would give me the opportunity to go beyond my ego state, opening the door to a new fascinating world, my "inner-world." What a great opportunity for the development or growth of my own soul!

Finally I understood that mirrors gave me information about me as a whole and that information was manifested through messages that were connecting my mind, body, and soul. For this reason mirrors became an essential part of my life, helping me to develop the idea of the Mirror Therapy, a routine that would help me to recover the balance in my life—a routine that was pure therapy for me!

Chapter 2

"The person who after having been careless, becomes attentive, illuminates the earth like the moon emerging from the clouds."
  Buddha

Losing Our Will

When we allow outside circumstances to interfere or block our free will, our power of intention disappears, we are alienated, and we become slaves to the outside—totally blind and out of control, like empty bodies going wherever life takes us. Once we are trapped we seek desperately for things that can restore the balance in our lives, but we do it unconsciously. We are so vulnerable and eager to try everything in a desperate way that we can fall easily into all kinds of addictions or mistaken behaviors. We are so blind that we are looking for answers in the wrong places, in the outside, forgetting completely that everything is occurring within and that the cure, the answer to our prayers, is right inside us.

It is really sad to see people trapped in the quest for physical perfection, desperate to change their outsides and completely lost, not knowing who they are anymore. Unfortunately we are living in a very materialistic society where it is so easy to lose the connection with our souls. Our lives are organized in such way that we forget completely how to take care of our inner selves. It seems like so many people are trapped in a meaningless world with no identity, being controlled by external factors that make them miserable and overwhelmed. A clear example of this is our daily newspapers, magazines, and TV programs showing us people's lives full of stress, worry, irritability, and anger, with no purpose in life, no power, no interest in living—just a profound sense of frustration.

We have to be honest and accept that our happiness can't be found in the material world in the "out-side." We have to liberate ourselves and stop being controlled by other beings and forces but rather control our own acts and thoughts. It is time to discover the real being inside; the real "self," this unique, lasting identity; the source of our thoughts, actions, and emotions—an identity that should remain the same through life.

I hope this book can help you out to recover your freedom and to understand that the beauty of life is feeling great from the inside out; it is balance connecting mind, body, and spirit; it is celebrating the uniqueness of life, knowing that we do have the most incredible gift: we have been given "will power." Once we understand that we have the power of choice our lives will be transformed completely. We will be connected to our higher selves, trusting our inner wisdom and finally discovering our real purpose in life. It will be the beginning of an incredible and meaningful life!

Chapter 3

"Better than a thousand meaningless words is a single sensible word, which can bring calm to the one who listens to it."
  Buddha

Transforming Lives

I had the privilege to study what I consider my passion, psychology. Since I can remember I have been fascinated by and interested in knowing more about our selves. I always wanted to understand human behavior, and I was concerned with generating explanations for the actions I observed.

I studied psychology at the University of Saint Thomas in Bogotá, Colombia. I graduated in 1993, and since then I have been focused on my professional goal of "helping people." I love applying my knowledge to human problems and giving someone in need hope, making his or her life a little bit easier. I know that it does not matter where I am or where I go, I always can help, and that makes me feel fulfilled and happy.

My professional position is based on humanistic-existential perspectives, a position that focuses on the uniqueness of individuals and a belief that they should be free to make their own choices about the directions they want to take in their own lives.

They should be allowed the opportunity to organize and control their own behavior.

I believe that as human beings we do have the right to develop our fullest potential of being creative and happy, looking inside ourselves and developing personal growth and respect for the worth of the individual and his or her innate potential. We have to understand that we are autonomous beings with the power to control our lives instead of being continually controlled by others or by circumstances.

Besides the traditional background I have in psychology, I have always been interested in holistic living, a different approach to life which teaches us how to discover and maintain natural homeostatic balance of mind, body, and spirit. My interest was so deep that I decided to study and learn more about it. After doing some research I found what I was looking for, the perfect match for my career, based on my principles and my interest in helping to bring others to health, happiness, and well being. I decided to study Healtheology. Healtheologists learn that at any level of being, each soul has a threefold purpose: to experience, learn, and express itself. Health-theology is a theological science of health exposing that the two share essential common ground; that successfully blending health with theology can indeed yield a sum that is far greater than its parts.

Those seeking relief from a specific condition can learn to recognize long-term good health as a rightful expectation, not the short-term conditions of ill health that they may temporarily experience. Theology, the study of God and divine law, is a science that affects human health to the extent to which we human beings are functioning in harmony with the universe based on our individual levels of awareness and our own thought processes.

I do really think that alternative therapies are helping so many people to take control of their lives, turning them back to more natural solutions to their problems. I definitely agree with some of the principles of these alternative therapies, which are rooted in ancient cultures, such as Chinese, Indian, Tibetan, African, and Native American cultures. Many alternative therapies define

The Mirror Therapy

health as balance within the body. Imbalance is thought to cause disease. The focus is on treating the whole person—physically, emotionally, mentally, and spiritually—so that balance can be restored. When balance is restored, the body can heal itself. In alternative medicine, health is also thought to be influenced by a person's experiences, environment, diet, and relationships with other people. This type of approach is called holistic.

Finally, as a human being I have been enriched with all kinds of experiences, and I have learned that everything that happens to us is for our good, even if what happens is painful. I know that my learning process is not finished yet. I believe that I have many lessons to learn in the school of life, but somehow I feel that at this point of my life I'm prepared to help others through education, sharing the knowledge I have gotten through professional and personal experiences.

Through education we develop the power of thinking, increasing our ability to search for personal worth, contributing to our self-realization, and ultimately contributing to the realization of our society. I believe that with knowledge we get power, and with power comes responsibility, and that's why I feel responsible, because through education we can prevent and relieve so many problems that are affecting our society.

Chapter 4

"If a person speaks or acts with a pure mind, then happiness follows, like the shadow that never leaves him."
    Buddha

Inspiring You

After many years of professional and personal growth, I decided to share my knowledge with all those people who are looking for a big change in their lives but do not know where to start or where to find the right answer. I want them to know that there is hope, that their lives are not over, that like me they can fight back, not giving up their dreams. I want to share my own personal experience with people to show them that no matter who you are or what you do, you can be trapped, too, and escape at the same time, because that's exactly what happened to me. I thought that as professional, as a psychologist, I was immune to these emotional and spiritual crises. I thought I had the knowledge to live a well-balanced life until I experienced what I consider the most difficult test of my life, an experience that changed completely my perspective about my profession and my personal beliefs. This change was so dramatic and so positive at the same time that I knew that sooner or later I had the responsibility to share it with people in emotional need.

Marcela Insignares

I want to use my personal experience as an example to guide you in your development as a human being because I truly believe that we learn not just from our experiences, but from the experiences of others, too. How we cope with our personal crises can inspire others! If someone can relate to my experience or my story and change his or her perspective about life in a positive way, I will accomplished my mission. My intention is to show you an example of will power inspiring you to change the circumstances that are interfering with the evolution of your soul.

Chapter 5

"Life is not a problem to be solved, but a reality to be experienced."
  Buddha

My Story, The Foundation of the Mirror Therapy

A few years ago my husband had the opportunity to work in the U.S.A., and we decided that it was time to experience something new and exciting. It was a good opportunity, and we definitely had to take advantage of it. The situation in my country, Colombia, was really bad, and violence was part of our lives. We thought that it was better to give our children the chance to live in a safer place and to have a better life.

Once we were in the United States, our situation was really hard as we were trying to survive in a different culture without family or friends. My husband was working full time and I had to stay at home taking care of my two boys. My life had changed completely. I realized that I did not have my mom to give me advice when I needed it most or a dad to spoil me, or my little sister to have fun with, or my brother to fight with. I had left everything, my friends, my job as a psychologist, my life in my country, which was not really bad at all. In my mind I was clear that it was time to grow, that I had my own family and I had to make sacrifices if I wanted a better life.

Marcela Insignares

I wanted to have everything under control and I really felt prepared for this big change in my life, but for some reason I started to feel things that I had never expected. At the beginning I thought it was "normal" to feel depressed, lonely, or anxious—it was just part of the process of adaptation. I did not realize that something really bad was happening to me, but slowly my emotions and feelings spiraled out of control. I was feeling completely lost and no longer capable physically and emotionally of living a "normal' or balanced life, and although I was trying really hard to rationalize my situation, I could not bear it anymore, ending up at the emergency room.

I remember that day like it was yesterday. Everything started one morning when I felt chest pain and a weird feeling in my body. I wanted to ignore it, but I started to experience other symptoms that really scared me, like palpitations, shortness of breath, and dizziness. I thought that what I was experiencing was a heart attack. I panicked and called my husband immediately; I told him that I had to go the hospital—that it was my heart and I needed help. It was the scariest and the longest day of my life; every second was an eternity. When my husband was driving to the hospital I was in complete shock, thinking that I was going to die. I thought that it was unfair. I was just twenty-seven years old with two small babies. I did not want to die, I wanted to take care of my children, I wanted to live! Once we got to hospital I remember the emergency room nurse asking me many questions, but I was so overwhelmed and confused that it was almost impossible to talk to her. I really did not want to talk—I just wanted to be saved!

After many questions and physical tests, the doctor came and explained the situation to me. I cannot forget his words: "You have just had a panic attack." I could not believe it. It was impossible—a psychologist having a panic attack! I refused to believe him, and I wanted a second opinion. I was almost sure that I had a heart condition, but after a valium and some rest, I understood that it was the truth. I was suffering from anxiety, a condition that I used to treat as professional but that I never

The Mirror Therapy

thought I was going to experience myself. I felt for the first time that my knowledge was just theory. All those years studying and treating anxiety disorders did not help me to recognize my own problems. I felt that I was not going to be able to help anybody anymore—including myself!

After a few months of darkness, one day I decided that I was not going to give up and it was time to apply my knowledge as professional to my own problems. I was in a position to derive some personal benefit from my career. Nobody was around to help me—I had no family, no friends, no money to pay a therapist, no insurance. The only thing I had at that point was my motivation, the desire in my heart to feel better, and the knowledge I had obtained through education and some personal and professional experiences. It was time to develop my own plan of action!

I realized that I had to develop my own therapy, something that could give me exactly what I needed based on my needs and circumstances. First it was crucial to understand my situation. I really had to know if I had a physical or mental condition that I needed to treat or if it was something else of which I was not aware. I think it is very important to recognize and evaluate the problems in our lives. I believe that we have to be conscious of our situation, being aware of the kind of life we are living. In my opinion that's the first step to recovery!

I never thought I was going to have a panic attack in my life, but for some reason I had to experience it. It changed me completely, professionally and personally. First of all, as professional, I experienced a condition I used to treat when I was practicing psychology in Colombia. I remember some patients describing their feelings when they were having panic attacks, and I remember my effort to understand what they were saying. It is hard to understand what a person feels when we have not experienced it ourselves. After I had a panic attack I understood exactly what those people were feeling. I was getting my lesson in a way that seemed ironic to me, because I had all these theories in my head, but for some reason it was not enough. I had to experience it myself to understand it. I learned the hard way, but I consider that lesson the most important lesson of my life. Professionally speaking, this experience has helped me to connect to people who suffer from anxiety disorders more easily.

Personally, I understood that no matter who we are or what we do, we are all humans, and that makes us vulnerable to all kinds of physical and mental conditions.

In my effort to understand my situation, the first step was to know more about anxiety and panic attacks. I had to spend a lot time doing research about anxiety disorders. I really needed to have more knowledge. When we know what it is happening to us, we can fight it and recover more easily. Remember, this is my experience and I have a professional background in mental health; if you suffer from any mental or physical condition, you should ask for professional advice. My purpose is to give you an example; it is not my intention to encourage you to diagnose or treat any mental or physical condition.)

After I reviewed a lot of books about anxiety, I confirmed that I had had some of the symptoms, like the period of intense fear or discomfort in the absence of real danger accompanied by somatic symptoms including palpitations, sweating, shaking, shortness of breath, and chest pain. I realized that my symptoms were unexpected; there was no association with an internal or external trigger. At that point I got really confused, because with no association to any internal or external trigger it was so difficult to determine the cause of these attacks.

Continuing with my research I decided to make an appointment with a doctor and discuss my situation. I really wanted to make sure I did not have a physical condition and see if there was something that could prevent me to experience another attack. After a complete physical examination, the doctor concluded that I had nothing to be worried about physically speaking, and like many other people I just had high levels of "stress." He said that if I wanted I could try some pills to reduce my levels of anxiety or maybe live a "less stressful life." (I did not tell him I was a psychologist. I wanted to be treated like any

The Mirror Therapy

regular patient with no knowledge about mental health. I did not want to contaminate the consultation.)

It was the first time I had spoken with a physician about my condition, and I wanted to explore a little bit more the medical approach to anxiety. Although I knew I did not have an extreme problem, I decided to take the pills and experience the effect on my body and my behavior. I had mixing feelings about this. I knew that I did not want any kind of pills to manipulate my mental patterns because I do really believe that drugs should be used except in extreme cases, but at the same time I wanted to experience myself the difference in my mind and body under the influence of this prescription. I wanted to try different things; I wanted to explore and educate myself it was part of my learning process.

The first day I took my medication I felt really nervous. It was like I was going to lose control of my life, but I was conscious that I had to try it if I wanted to know the effects. I felt really weird, completely numb. I could not drive, and I did not have energy to do anything. It was like I was floating, unable to catch the rhythm of life, and it was my first day.

I gave up! It was definitely not for me. One single pill was enough to understand that I had to face my problems, getting to the roots of them, and fight in a more "natural" way.

Thankfully I had experienced just three panic attacks in a period of seven years. It was not a considerable number to diagnose a panic disorder, however, I needed to know what was causing those attacks and why. If I did not have a panic disorder that I needed to treat as a mental condition, what was it? What was causing those symptoms? What was causing the anxiety? I had to investigate and get to the roots of my situation if I wanted to recover the balance I had lost. After I discarded the possibility of a physical or mental condition, I decided to change my focus and direct my attention to a different *holistic* approach. I had been always interested in this different approach to life, and I definitely agreed with some of its principles, so I thought that it was time to try something different and more meaningful to me.

Marcela Insignares

I decided to be more focused on myself, exploring my inner-world and connecting the main parts of my being: spirit, mind, and body. I was seeking for balanced, self-conscious awareness in order to live a healthier and happier life.

The result was unbelievable. My life was transformed completely, my symptoms disappeared, my balance was restored, and I felt better than ever.

It took me time and a lot of hard work to understand my situation. It was not an easy task to find what was hidden within, but finally I did.

I thought that as a professional psychologist I had the knowledge to understand human behavior. I was always trying to answer my questions with the rational mind, but with time I understood that sometimes these logical and rational deductions were very limited and without depth. It was crucial to explore my inner-self if I wanted to find the answers to my deepest questions.

After a lot of research and study about myself, I finally found what was happening to me. I concluded that what was causing my imbalance was the high level of anxiety that I was experiencing due to my effort to live a "perfect life."

I had become like many other people, a slave to the outside. I thought that my priority was to help everybody—family, friends, people in need—and I wanted to have everything under control. I wanted to be the perfect wife, the perfect mother, the perfect human being. Forgetting completely about myself, I ignored the being within, thinking that giving everything to the outside, to others, was enough to achieve my dreams and fulfill my life.

I allowed the circumstances to drive me until I could not resist anymore. I was consumed in the outside, living an unrealistic life and looking for physical perfection and egocentric goals that slowly were destroying my real self.

I believe that there are no coincidences, that things happen for a reason. That's why I can say that I was blessed when I became aware of the kind of life I was living, because I made conscious the feelings and emotions that were hidden within and which I was unaware of. Most importantly, it made me realize that I was a whole and I had to connect my body, mind, and soul if I wanted to live a peaceful, balanced, and happy life.

After I discovered the cause of my imbalance, I decided to create something that could help me to connect to my inner self more easily and keep me in great shape spiritually, physically, and mentally. I wanted a healthy habit, a routine or discipline just for me and designed by me. It was the beginning of *The Mirror Therapy!*

Chapter 6

"With our thoughts, we create the world."
Buddha

Developing the Mirror Therapy, Creating the Structure

Once I got consciousness of my situation, understanding that I had the responsibility to take care of myself, I decided to create something that could help me to connect to my higher self, something that would give me the opportunity to express my deepest feelings and emotions, being in control again, and something that definitely could help me to improve my quality of life.

I don't know how many books I read about psychology and self-help, plus spiritual growth and all kind of disciplines to learn how to live a better life. I learned about alternative medicine, yoga, Pilates, and so many things that could help me to recover the balance I had lost. It was overwhelming because I had a lot of information but I did not know how to use it, and there was always something new, something I wanted to try. I was going from one thing to another, not knowing exactly what I wanted and, the most important thing, what I really needed.

I wanted to try everything from heavy routines of exercise to meditation, but I did not know how to take advantage of each specific new thing I was trying. It seemed like nothing was really working. There was something missing. I was not really connecting myself with any of the alternatives that life was bringing me. At that point I realized that I had to personalize a routine or create a discipline because I really wanted something different and unique, something based on my own needs and circumstances. I did not want to be a blind follower anymore!

I saw for the first time the path to recovery, the light for which I was hoping. It was a long process and I really had to study a lot, but it was more than worth it!

I knew I had valuable information and a lot of knowledge which I had gotten through professional and personal experiences. I had everything I needed to develop what I was looking for. The first thing I did was to organize my thoughts, analyzing carefully every piece of information I had in my head and how it related to my situation. After that I abstracted what I considered could be the foundation of my routine, and using my imagination and creativity I developed the Mirror Therapy.

The Mirror Therapy had everything I needed and everything I wanted. It was my masterpiece, containing valuable concepts, elements, and techniques that I considered were the perfect combination to achieve the results I wanted. The entire process was the result of my quest for wholeness, it was the integration of the main parts of my being. I really had to connect my mind, spirit, and body to be able to develop it. All my knowledge, my emotions, and feelings were materialized through this experience. I had to go beyond my ego and discover the real person inside. There were no hidden messages anymore, no masks, no fear to explore.

Once I began the development of the Mirror Therapy, I started to understand the dynamic within and the amazing power that I had to transform my circumstances. For the first time I felt free to choose. My power of intention was back. My will power was back!

Remember, nobody can give us the answers that we want to hear. We cannot forget that we are unique, that every human being

The Mirror Therapy

has an essence, a soul, that can't be shared with anybody. That's why it is very important to have clear in your mind and in your heart what you really want and why.

I know now how powerful we are, and I think I'm a good example of someone who never gave up, someone who believed in a better life, and someone who was willing to do everything possible to achieve peace of mind. Through the development and practice of the Mirror Therapy, I learned that no matter how desperate we are there is always hope because we do have the power of self-transformation. God makes us creative, and we are the designers of our lives. We can make our own decisions because we have will power. It is our right to express ourselves freely and develop our fullest potential as human beings with a soul. That's the path to personal growth.

I can say proudly today that I am a happy human being. I feel stronger than ever physically, emotionally, and spiritually. My symptoms disappeared completely, and my balance was restored. I can go on and on telling you all the blessings that the Mirror Therapy has brought to my life, but now it is your time to experience it and bring the blessings to your life!

I'll show you step by step how to create your routine, and I hope you can use it as a guide to your learning process. I'll share with you what I consider the basic concepts, elements, and techniques that you can use as an example to develop your own routine, but remember that you are the creator and you should trust your own process, your own instincts, feeling free to experience all the things you want, exploring the unknown world of yourself. Don't forget that you possess an inner-guide system that will show you the right path to follow. Trust it; trust yourself. It is exactly what I did!

The Mirror Therapy is above all an adventure, one that involves inner work. It is for people who are really interested in creating their own discipline, routine, or therapy — the name is not important. What matter most is the objective, and I can say for sure that we all do have the same goal: to live great lives.

Part II
Creating Your Routine

Chapter 1
What Is the Real Meaning of the Mirror Therapy?

The Mirror Therapy is a journey of discovery and experience that is unique for each person. It is designed by you for you. You will find the right tools and techniques by which you may discern the best path to take in your life. You will be in control, feeling inspired and unleashing the power within, releasing all the negativity and finally finding peace.

The Mirror Therapy will make your existence a life-long learning venture. If you are patient and practice regularly, you will achieve the results you want. A commitment to regular practice is essential to master any discipline. Remember that you are the designer, that you possess all that is required to successfully develop your routine. You will experience the power of self-transformation, the power of intention, the power of will!

Believe in yourself, in your own capabilities, and working on your routine you will find the strength you need to live a great life. You believe, you trust, you wish, you make it possible!

Each individual decides for his or her own self how much effort to put into the routine, how much hard work, how much time and energy. You will go at your own speed, trusting your instincts, discovering what is best for you.

Love yourself. Love every moment of your experience, and you will find your journey full of beautiful surprises.

Marcela Insignares

If you decide to follow my routine as it is, you will find all the basic things that you need to be in balance, but if you think that there is something missing feel free to explore new possibilities. Be creative!

Chapter 2
The Elements

The elements are the basic things that you need to start your routine. They are simple but very important. Remember, you can add, change, or discover your own elements. Take my example as a guide and feel free to experience new things.

Mirrors

I've been always fascinated by mirrors. I think they can connect us to our higher selves; we just need to learn how to use them. If we discover their power we will have a great tool which allows us to reach our inner selves, giving us the opportunity to see who we really are. For this reason I chose mirrors as a tool.

I used to spend hours in front of mirrors trying to look better, fixing my hair or make-up or looking for defects to correct. It was torture sometimes. I had bad days and good days, and I could not understand why sometimes I looked so good and sometimes I looked so bad. After I studied myself deeply and I started the exploration of my inner world, I realized that mirrors were giving me information about my soul. It was not just my body looking good or bad, it was my soul trying to communicate with me through feelings, emotions, and expressions that before I could not understand.

Marcela Insignares

I started to pay attention to the reflection of my body, carefully thinking that there were hidden messages that I had to understand, messages that would help me to discover the real being I was. If you decide to follow the Mirror Therapy, it is very important to have a big mirror. You should be able to see the reflection of your entire body from head to toe. If you want you can use more than one mirror; you could create a circle of mirrors.

The idea is to be able to observe yourself from different perspectives.

The Zone

This is your place, a sacred place where everything is possible, where dreams come true, where there is no limitation to the self, where you make conscious all the feelings and emotions that are hidden within, and where you become a whole, connecting, and balancing soul, mind, and body. It is a place of peace and tranquility, somewhere you will be undisturbed, a space with no phones, no interruptions, just you willing to start the most incredible journey of your life. This place will put you in the right frame of mind to begin your routine.

Time

You have to decide how often you want to work on your routine. Be realistic about how much time you can give each week. Make your decision, then stick to it as much as possible. My advice is to set aside at least thirty minutes per routine, three times a week.

Inner knowing requires you to be fully present. For that reason it is important to get your spirit back into the here and now. This is the only way to make possible our self-exploration.

Clothing

Wear something that makes you feel good. Use whatever you want or are in the mood for. Experience new things, play with your clothes, use your imagination, but do not forget to be comfortable because your body will move spontaneously and uncomfortable clothes will limit your movement.

The Mirror Therapy

I love to see my body as it is. I'm not worried about my physical imperfection anymore; that's why I feel comfortable with little things or no clothes at all!

Music

Studies show that there are musical characteristics that affect our emotional state. We tend to have different emotional reactions to different kinds of music. We can feel sad, playful, happy, excited, or dreamy and spiritual. There is no doubt that we are deeply influenced by the music we like best!

You should do your homework and pick your favorite tapes or CDs. You will need a good selection or a variety of music, mixing different rhythms and lyrics. They will help you to feel motivated and energized. Music you like gives the best boost to your spiritual, mental and physical workout.

Remember, it is important to choose the right music to achieve the effect you want. Have fun collecting the music you like.

Chapter 3
The Techniques

At this point you have an example of different elements that you can use for your program, but you need to add techniques to complete the routine. I will provide you with a list of techniques that I developed based on traditional and alternative therapies. They are the backbone of the Mirror Therapy.

Do not forget that you can try these techniques and use them as a part of your program, or you can do some research and explore other possibilities.

Breathing

I do think that my breath is a mirror for my mind. Breath and mind are definitely connected. Any alteration in one will affect the other. Awareness of the breath will bring your mind to the present moment. Your breath is the monitor of how you are doing in the routine and in your life. Each person's breathing is unique, a personal experience that reflects how we feel inside and out. When we breathe better, we feel better, and conscious breathing is a powerful ally in life that provides a sense of well being.

Breath and movement are clearly linked so that you feel the flow. While you are doing your routine, bring constancy to your breath. When the breath flows steadily there will be a feeling of cleansing, lightness, balance, physical energy, and mental clarity.

Do experiment to intuit what feels right for your body. A good breathing habit is a valuable tool for self-management.

Self-talking

With some time and effort I realized that simple exercises could help us to communicate better to our inner selves. When I see the reflection of myself in the mirror, I am always looking for clues, asking myself different questions about the things I see. Why do I look sad today, or tired, or stressed out? How do I feel at this moment? Is there something that is bothering me? Why am I gaining too much weight? How can improve my situation? If we are honest in answering these simple questions, we will find a way to explore our inner world, going beyond our egos. With time we will train ourselves to go deeply, opening the door to this fascinating world within us. Believe me, you will be surprised by the results.

This technique allows us to have conversation with ourselves. Do not feel afraid of this self-talking. Do it aloud in front of your mirror; it plays a big role in the Mirror Therapy. You will reveal all the secrets that you have hidden; the only thing you need is honesty. It is important to be sincere. Remember, there is nobody around to judge you. Feel free to take off all the masks you wear in front of people. You will see the real being, going beyond the ego state. Simple questions like, Who am I? What is my purpose in my life? What should I do to be happy? Am I happy? will open your mind, and you will be able to go deeper, exploring yourself and finding the answers for which you were waiting.

Remember, you are the only one who can go inside and explore within. It is a unique experience. Nobody can do it for you, and although it seems a little difficult at the beginning, don't worry. It is just a matter of time. Be perseverant, and believe me, you will have the best friend you can have: *yourself*.

Affirmations

We know that affirmations help us to reinforce our hopes,

The Mirror Therapy

dreams, dignity, respect, and all the rights with which we were born.

Write a list of affirmations. Be creative, use your own words, follow your intuition, and put on paper what you consider the most powerful list of words in your life.

Read out loud this list of affirmations in front of your mirror. Feel every word, meaning what you are saying. Observe the expression on your face while you are reading. What do you see? What do you feel?

With time you will memorize these affirmations and you will be able to use them anytime. Feel empowered and encouraged to bring to reality what you say. Thoughts are powerful!

Visualization

Most people are familiar with this term. It is very common these days and is part of many programs. In my case, I had to personalize this important technique because I knew that it was going to be very helpful.

My goal was to explore facets of myself that I had never before explored. I wanted to encounter other realities which could take me to a higher level of understanding I never dreamed possible. To me, visualization is being able to create in the mind a scene, a situation, or an experience. It is playing with my imagination, feeling that there is no limitation to the self.

When I am in front of my mirror I pay close attention to my reflection, and using my imagination I visualize the things I want in my life. Visualization gives you the opportunity to do whatever you want. You can travel and see yourself in different situations, or if you are afraid of something or someone this is a great opportunity to face your fears. Do not limit yourself!

Visualization is really a liberating experience. Do not be surprised if you discover that hidden within you resides someone very talented with abilities that were previously unknown. Go ahead and have fun dreaming, because you never know if your dreams will come true someday.

Self-expression

Although the other techniques are important, I consider this one the most powerful of my routine because it helped me to express myself in a way I never thought possible.

Self-expression as a technique means to give permission to myself to do whatever I feel in a moment; it means freedom to express myself with no fear of judgment.

I remember when I was little and I used to pretend in front of the mirror that I was a singer or a dancer. I used to spend a lot time in my room dreaming about being someone important, and using my imagination I created different realities that allowed me to transport myself to places I never dreamt of. What a great feeling!

I think these memories of my childhood helped me to develop this technique. I wanted to experience this feeling of freedom again, dreaming and expressing through my body all the emotions I had inside. I really wanted to bring out the child within; I wanted to feel liberated and happy; I wanted to dream again!

While I was developing this technique I discovered that with music and movement I could bring out emotions and feelings that were hidden within. It was easier to open my mind and feel motivated to explore different realities. I knew that I had found the best way to release all the energy and vitality I had.

I truly believe that music makes us happier and more motivated, and movement allows us to release energy through our body — besides we can express ourselves in a way we really enjoy. It is pure therapy, a liberating experience, and it is really fun.

First of all you need to get motivated. For that reason you must choose your favorite music. This is very important. You will need a variety of CDs or tapes mixing different rhythms and lyrics to which you can relate. You will use them according to the way you feel or your mood.

Once you have your favorite music, you will allow yourself to express freely through movement. You do not have to be in perfect shape or physical condition because this is not a routine of exercise. It is just your getting to know and control your body in a better way. You will go at your own pace, discovering the inner

The Mirror Therapy

rhythm. It is part of the self-exploration you are doing and a great way to connect mind, body, and soul.

You will feel a little shy at the beginning, but believe me, with time you will be a master. Do not be afraid to do all the things you want. Feel free to express yourself, dancing, singing, moving all your body in a way you never before experienced — but don't forget to do it in front of your mirror. You will get to see your body from a different perspective, getting new information about yourself, exploring new facets, and finally being in tune with the universe.

Remember, use the imagination and play. This is your time!

Integration/Liberation: Where Everything Converges

The ultimate goal of the Mirror Therapy is create a moment where everything converges: the elements, the techniques, and of course, the being. Observe the reflection of yourself in the mirror, see the way you move and control your body, pay attention to every single part, talk to yourself. Express what you are feeling at that particular moment, bringing yourself to the present, experiencing the power of now. Do not feel afraid of anything, because you are in control. You will discover the way to bring out feelings and emotions that are within you but for whatever reason have not been expressed.

Relaxation

You will center yourself, allowing your body to integrate and consolidate the effects of the routine you have been doing.

I use yoga relaxation, which allows me to bring my body, mind, and spirit back into balance. After a strong session where I really have explored my boundaries, this active undoing comes more easily. I take a break from vigorous external movement and lie perfectly still. While I progressively let go of tension in the muscles, bones, internal organs, and even the brain, I remain aware of the internal sensations.

Whenever your thoughts stray, bring them back to your body. Physically and mentally permit yourself to release all negativity, being just you, nothing else, lying on the floor. Relaxation is a good preparation for meditation.

Meditation

Meditation is a very deeply personal experience. In meditation we practice to be the observer, not the doer. Through meditation you will detach yourself from negative feelings and thoughts, developing a deeper understanding of who you are and who you may become. You will have a different perspective about life.

When I meditate I just sit quietly, turning my attention inward toward a specific subject. I observe my thoughts and remain detached, without altering the thought patterns at all. This is a great way to develop my awareness, in other words, the capacity to notice fully every event in my life as it happens.

For many people relaxation and meditation can be really difficult tasks. I gave you an idea of how to achieve these two states of mind, but you have to discover by yourself which is the best way to get the results you want. In my case I used yoga exercises based on information I got through books and I practiced for a long period of time, but remember that there is not a perfect point. Although we can use information as a guide, we have to trust our inner-guide system. I truly believe that we do have the capacity to discern what is best for us. We just need to listen to our inner voice; it will be the best guidance!

Chapter 4
Benefits

You will notice the effects on your life from following your routine. It will take time, but with patience and discipline the results will be amazing.

Some of the benefits you can experience are that you will begin to mold your attitude, change your perspective on life, be more positive, and finally give healing to yourself. The whole process will help you to be more joyful, more at peace.

The mirror therapy is a journey of discovery and experience that is unique for each person. You will be the seeker of your own truth, challenging your understanding of life, giving yourself a sense of spiritual renewal.

You will be able to discern the best path to take in your life among several choices. You will be in charge of your life, making plans for your journey through this school of life.

You will feel more beautiful than ever, understanding that God created us beautiful, that our human body is the temple where the soul resides. No matter what shape it takes, you will appreciate it.

You will develop a healthy habit which will bring out the best in you, feeling inspired, creative, and more powerful than ever, with no limitations; feeling capable of achieving all the dreams you have in a way you never before thought possible.

Marcela Insignares

The discipline that you will develop is a mind-body-spirit workout. Through movement you will engage your body, mind, and spirit, releasing negative thoughts, bringing out emotions and feelings you were not aware of, promoting harmony and balance.

You will be able to explore yourself, discovering fascinating information that you will use to develop your soul.

The Mirror Therapy will benefit you as a whole person. It promotes physical relaxation and calm, reducing stress and anxiety in your life. You can find peace of mind by learning to detach yourself from negative or troubling thoughts.

You will transform your experience day by day, wiping out your fears, crossing limitations, and bringing more joy and peace to each moment.

Once you find the point of equilibrium, the real balance within, you will not have the feeling of hurting yourself anymore. Thoughts of auto-destructive behavior will disappear completely.

You will realize that, being human, you are allowed to make mistakes. You will learn not to regret past actions; you will learn from them.

You will consciously choose to accept responsibility for being the person you are, recognizing that you and only you are in charge of your life.

This list can go on and on. You will discover more and more benefits along the journey. I hope you can open your heart and be prepared to receive all the blessings that this simple but powerful discipline will give you. Good Luck!

Chapter 5
My Favorite Quotes

I would like to share with you my favorite quotes which I collected through the development of my project. I think they are instructive and entertaining statements that are full of wisdom.

I used to eat in my favorite Chinese restaurant and I loved to read the fortune cookies given to me each time I was there. My favorites are:

> Your destiny lies before you, choose wisely.
> We should not expect from others
>   what we cannot do ourselves.
> Keep in mind your most cherished dreams of the future.
> Fortune truly helps those who are of good judgment.
> Good sense is the master of human life.

Other quotes:

> Happiness resides
> not in possessions
> and not in gold;
> the feeling of happiness
> dwells in the soul.
>   Democritus

Marcela Insignares

My respect for individuals is a respect for their right to be, to live, to explore their own potentialities, to find their own salvation, to achieve what dignity they can. It is not an indiscriminate enthusiasm for the general level of human performance. Great talent and the high virtues are thinly dispersed and no intensity of democratic sentiment will change the fact.
    D. Sutten

The best part of one's life is the working part, the creative part. Believe me I love to succeed...However, the real spiritual and emotional excitement is in the doing.
    Garson Kanin

Any man may play his part in the mummery, and act the honest man on the scaffolding; but to be right within, in his own bosson, where all is allowed, where all is concealed -- there's the point! The next step is to be so in our own home, in our ordinary actions, of which we need render no account to any man, where there is no study, no make believe.
    Montaigne

Education is a companion which no misfortune can depress, no crime can destroy, no enemy can alienate, no despotism can slave. At home a friend, abroad an introduction, in solitude a solace, and in society an ornament. It chastens vice, it guides virtue, it gives, at once, grace and government to genius. Without it, what is man? A splendid slave, a reasoning savage.
    Joseph Addison

The most beautiful and most profound emotion we can experience is the sensation of the mystical. It is the dower of all true science. He to whom this emotion is a stranger, who can no longer wonder

and stand rapt in awe, is as good as dead. To know that was impenetrable to us really exists, manifesting itself as the highest wisdom and the most radiant beauty which our dull faculties can comprehend only in their most primitive forms—this knowledge, this feeling is at the center of true religiousness.
    Albert Einstein

God does not die on the day when we cease to believe in a personal deity, but we die on the day when our lives cease to be illuminated by the steady radiance, renewed daily, of a wonder, the source of which is beyond all reason.
    Dag Hammarskjold

Existence is a strange bargain. Life owes little; we owe it everything. The only true happiness comes from squandering ourselves for a purpose.
    John Mason Brown

This is the true joy in life, the being used for a purpose recognized by yourself as a mighty one; the being thoroughly worn out before you are thrown on the scrap heap; the being a force of Nature instead of a feverish, selfish little clod of ailments and grievances complaining that the world will not devote itself to making you happy.
    George Bernard Shaw

. . . Many have but one resource to sustain them in their misery, and that is to think, "circumstances have been against me... I have never had a great love...but that is because I have never met a man or a woman...worthy of it; if I had not written ...good books, it is because I had not the leisure."... But...for the existentialist, there is no love apart from deeds of love; no potentiality of love other than that which is manifested in loving; there is no genius other than

Marcela Insignares

that which is expressed in works of art.
    Jean Paul Sartre

The more faithfully you listen to the voice within you, the better you will hear what is sounding outside. And only he who listens can speak.
    Dag Hammarskjold

I care not so much what I am to others as I respect what I am in myself. I will be rich by myself and not by borrowing.
    Montaigne

There is a light that shines beyond all things on earth, beyond us all, beyond the heavens, beyond the highest, the very highest heavens. This is the light that shines in our hearth.
    Chandogya Upanishad

Though words are spoken to explain the void,
The void as such can never be expressed.
Though we say, "the mind is a bright light,"
It is beyond all words and symbols.
Although the mind is void in essence,
All things it embraces and contains.
    Tilopa
    The Song of Hahahudra

Thine own consciousness, shining, void, and inseparable from the great body of radiance,
hath no birth, nor death, and is the Immutable Boundless Light.
    Padmasambhava
    The Tibetan Book of Death

The Mirror Therapy

It is not weeds that choke out the grain,
it is the negligence of the farmer.
    Confucius

Wisdom is not meditation on death, but on life.
    Spinoza

The faults of others are easy to see;
Our own are hard to see.
    Buddha

The world is blind. Rare are those who see.
    Buddha

Life is like a story. What is important is not how long it is, but how good it is.
    Seneca

The knowledge that is not supplemented
daily decreases every day.
    Chinese proverb

Do not be afraid of being slow,
only of stooping.
    Confucius

With time and patience,
the leaf of the mulberry tree becomes silk.
    Chinese proverb

References

American Institute of Holistic Theology, Inc. catalog. 2004.

Beers, Mark H., ed. *The Merck Manual of Health and Aging*. Whitehouse Station, NJ: Merck & Co., Inc., 2004. 52–53.

Brown, Christina. *The Book of Yoga*. Bath, UK: Parragon Publishing, 2002.

Desbois, Hervé. *Being Zen*. Loval, Quebec, Canada: Modus Vivendi Publishing Inc., 2001.

Gardner, John W. and Francesca Gardner Reese. *Quotations of With and Wisdom*. New York: W.W. Norton & Co., Inc., 1996.

Gray, Alex. *The Sacred Mirrors: The Visionary Art of Alex Grey with Essays by Ken Wilber, Carlo McCormick, Alex Grey*. Rochester, VT: Inner Traditions International, 1990.

Quotations are from Roger Lipsey's *An Art of Our Own* (Boston: Shambala Publications, 1988) See also, *The Spiritual in Art -- Abstract Art 1890-1985* (New York: Abbeville Press, 1986).